Charcot Marie Tooth Disease

A Beginner's Quick Start Guide to Managing CMT Through Diet, With Sample Curated Recipes

mf

copyright © 2022 Patrick Marshwell

All rights reserved No part of this book may be reproduced, or stored in a retrieval system, or transmitted in any form or by any means, electronic, mechanical, photocopying, recording, or otherwise, without express written permission of the publisher.

Disclaimer

By reading this disclaimer, you are accepting the terms of the disclaimer in full. If you disagree with this disclaimer, please do not read the guide.

All of the content within this guide is provided for informational and educational purposes only, and should not be accepted as independent medical or other professional advice. The author is not a doctor, physician, nurse, mental health provider, or registered nutritionist/dietician. Therefore, using and reading this guide does not establish any form of a physician-patient relationship.

Always consult with a physician or another qualified health provider with any issues or questions you might have regarding any sort of medical condition. Do not ever disregard any qualified professional medical advice or delay seeking that advice because of anything you have read in this guide. The information in this guide is not intended to be any sort of medical advice and should not be used in lieu of any medical advice by a licensed and qualified medical professional.

The information in this guide has been compiled from a variety of known sources. However, the author cannot attest to or guarantee the accuracy of each source and thus should not be held liable for any errors or omissions.

You acknowledge that the publisher of this guide will not be held liable for any loss or damage of any kind incurred as a result of this guide or the reliance on any information provided within this guide. You acknowledge and agree that you assume all risk and responsibility for any action you undertake in response to the information in this guide.

Using this guide does not guarantee any particular result (e.g., weight loss or a cure). By reading this guide, you acknowledge that there are no guarantees to any specific outcome or results you can expect.

All product names, diet plans, or names used in this guide are for identification purposes only and are the property of their respective owners. The use of these names does not imply endorsement. All other trademarks cited herein are the property of their respective owners.

Where applicable, this guide is not intended to be a substitute for the original work of this diet plan and is, at most, a supplement to the original work for this diet plan and never a direct substitute. This guide is a personal expression of the facts of that diet plan.

Where applicable, persons shown in the cover images are stock photography models and the publisher has obtained the rights to use the images through license agreements with third-party stock image companies.

Table of Contents

Introduction   6
What Causes Charcot-Marie-Tooth Disease?   8
   What are the genetic factors that cause CMT disease?   8
What Are the Symptoms of Charcot-Marie-Tooth Disease?   10
How Is Charcot-Marie-Tooth Disease Diagnosed?   13
   Who is at risk of getting CMT disease?   15
What Are the Complications of CMT Disease?   17
How to Manage Charcot-Marie-Tooth Disease Through Diet and Nutrition?   21
   Foods to Eat   21
   Foods to Avoid   27
Sample Recipes   29
   Vegan Caribbean Bowl   30
   Baked Flounder   32
   Salmon with Avocados and Brussels Sprouts   33
   Kale Fried Rice   36
   Asian-Themed Macrobiotic Bowl   38
   Chicken Salad   40
   Baked Salmon   41
   Asian Zucchini Salad   42
   Low FODMAP Burger   43
   Stir-Fried Cabbage and Apples   44
   Asparagus and Greens Salad with Tahini and Poppy Seed Dressing   45
   Stir-Fried Cabbage and Apples   46
Managing CMT Through Lifestyle and Natural Methods   47
Conclusion   49
FAQ About Charcot-Marie-Tooth Disease   50
References and Helpful Links   53

Introduction

The term "Charcot-Marie-Tooth disease," usually abbreviated as "CMT," refers to a group of inherited conditions that affect the nerves in the extremities and can lead to nerve damage.

Jean-Martin Charcot, Pierre Marie, and Howard Henry Tooth were the physicians who originally characterized the sickness in 1886. The condition was given their names in honor of their contributions. According to mda.org, there are around 19 cases of CMT for every 100,000 persons who are part of the general population.

CMT is distinguished by the gradual deterioration of muscular strength and atrophy, as well as a loss of sensation in the extremities, particularly the hands and feet. The symptoms of CMT normally start appearing in childhood or adolescence, and the condition typically advances gradually throughout one's lifetime.

However, some treatments can help to reduce symptoms and slow the progression of the condition. Although there is no cure for CMT at this time, there are treatments available.

With the assistance of various assistive technology and adaptive equipment, some people who have CMT can live lives that are close to normal. Diet and nutrition are also very significant factors to consider while trying to alleviate the symptoms of CMT.

In this beginner's guide, we'll cover the following in detail:

- What causes Charcot-Marie-tooth disease?
- What are the genetic factors that Cause CMT Disease?
- What are the symptoms of Charcot-Marie-tooth disease?
- How is Charcot-Marie-tooth disease diagnosed?
- Who is at risk to get Charcot-Marie-tooth disease?
- What are the complications of Charcot-Marie-Tooth disease?
- How to manage Charcot-Marie-tooth disease through diet and nutrition?
- Managing CMT through natural methods and lifestyle changes.

So, let's get started!

What Causes Charcot-Marie-Tooth Disease?

Mutations in genes that are responsible for the formation and maintenance of the peripheral nervous system are the root cause of CMT. Myelin, the protective sheath that covers nerve fibers, is lost as a result of these abnormalities. Because of this damage, the nerves become more vulnerable to further injury, which ultimately results in the symptoms that are diagnostic of CMT.

In addition, CMT can be inherited from one generation to the next since the mutations that cause it can be handed down from parent to child. This is because CMT is an inherited disorder.

What are the genetic factors that cause CMT disease?

CMT is not caused by a single bad gene. Different gene changes cause different kinds of CMT, and the bad genes can be passed down in several ways. A person with CMT may have gotten the genetic flaw that causes the condition from just one parent or both.

Autosomal dominant pattern

In this pattern, one parent has CMT and passes the mutated gene to the child. The child then has a one-half chance of passing the mutated gene on to his or her children.

Autosomal recessive pattern

In this pattern, both parents must have the mutated gene for the child to inherit it. If just one parent has the mutated gene, the child will not have CMT. However, the child will be a carrier of the mutated gene and can pass it on to his or her children.

X-linked pattern

This type of CMT is caused by mutations in genes on the X chromosome. The X chromosome is one of the two sex chromosomes. Females have two X chromosomes, while males have one X chromosome and one Y chromosome. This means that males are more likely to inherit X-linked CMT from their mothers. Females are less likely to inherit the condition, but they can still pass on the mutated gene to their children.

What Are the Symptoms of Charcot-Marie-Tooth Disease?

The symptoms of CMT vary depending on the type and severity of the disease. However, common symptoms include:

Muscle weakness

Weakness in the muscles is one of the most common symptoms of Charcot-Marie-Tooth disease. In most cases, the symptoms first appear in the muscles of the hands, feet, and legs. Weakness in the muscles can range from mild to severe, and it may get worse over time as the condition gets worse.

Muscle atrophy

Muscle atrophy is a common symptom of Charcot-Marie-Tooth disease. This degenerative disorder causes nerve damage and muscle weakness. As the disease progresses, muscles begin to waste away. This can lead to paralysis and loss of sensation in the limbs.

In severe cases, it can also affect the respiratory muscles, making it difficult to breathe. Muscle atrophy is often visible as a decrease in muscle mass and a loss of muscle definition. It can also cause joint pain and deformities.

Loss of sensation

One symptom of Charcot-Marie-Tooth Disease is loss of sensation. This can present itself in several ways, including numbness or tingling in the extremities, loss of proprioception (the ability to sense the positioning of one's limbs), and muscle weakness.

Loss of sensation can make everyday activities difficult or even impossible to perform. For example, someone with a loss of proprioception may have difficulty walking, as they are unable to sense where their feet are on the ground. In severe cases, loss of sensation can lead to paralysis.

Pain

One of the less common symptoms of Charcot-Marie-Tooth Disease is unexplained pain. While the individual suffering may feel pain in different parts of their body, it is most commonly experienced in the hands and feet. The pain can be described as a burning or tingling sensation and is often worse at night.

Though the pain can be intermittent, it can also be constant. For some people, the pain is mild and only causes discomfort. However, for others, the pain can be severe and debilitating. Treatment for this symptom typically includes pain medications, physical therapy, and orthopedic devices. In some cases, surgery may also be necessary. If you are experiencing unexplained pain, it is important to speak to your doctor to rule out other potential causes.

Fatigue

Fatigue is another common symptom of CMTD, as the muscles are not receiving the necessary signals from the brain to function properly. The fatigue can be mild or severe, and it can often be exacerbated by physical activity. As a result, people with CMTD often find it difficult to participate in activities that they once enjoyed.

How Is Charcot-Marie-Tooth Disease Diagnosed?

Charcot-Marie-Tooth disease is diagnosed through a combination of clinical observations and genetic testing. The symptoms of the disease can vary from person to person, so it is important to have a thorough evaluation by a healthcare professional.

Physical Exam

A Charcot-Marie-Tooth disease physical exam looks for muscle weakness and atrophy. In Charcot-Marie-Tooth Disease, there is a loss of nerve cells in the arms and legs. This loss results in muscle weakness and atrophy. The physical exam may also look for sensory loss.

The examiner will assess the strength of the muscles and the level of sensation in the extremities. The Charcot-Marie-Tooth disease physical exam can help to determine the severity of the condition and may be used to monitor the progression of the disease.

Electromyography

Electromyography (EMG) and nerve conduction studies are used to measure the function of motor neurons and the nerves that supply them. These tests can help diagnose Charcot-Marie-Tooth Disease (CMT) by identifying abnormalities in the electrophysiological signals that are sent from the brain to the muscles.

EMG records the electrical activity of muscles at rest and during contraction, while nerve conduction studies measure how well and how fast electrical signals are conducted through nerves. Both of these tests can help to reveal problems with the structure or function of nerve fibers, which can then be used to diagnose CMT. In some cases, EMG and nerve conduction studies may also be used to determine the severity of CMT and to monitor disease progression.

Genetic test

A genetic test may be conducted to look for mutations in the genes that are known to cause CMT. This test can help to confirm a diagnosis of CMT, and it can also be used to predict which family members are at risk of developing the disease. In some cases, a genetic test may also be used to guide treatment decisions.

Who is at risk of getting CMT disease?

CMT is a hereditary disorder that primarily affects the peripheral nerves. CMT runs in families, and those who have a family history of the condition are more likely to get it.

CMT may also be induced by spontaneous changes in DNA. This implies that anybody can get CMT even if there isn't a family history of the condition.

Family history of CMT

If you have a family member with CMT, you're at a higher risk of developing the condition. This is because CMT is often passed down from generation to generation.

Having a family member with CMT doesn't guarantee that you'll develop the condition, but it does increase your risk. If you're concerned about your risk, speak to your doctor or a genetic counselor.

No family history of CMT

CMT can also happen when a new mutation happens during pregnancy. These are called spontaneous mutations, and after they happen, they can be passed on to the next generation.

Spontaneous mutations are thought to account for a small minority of CMT cases, but they may be responsible for some of the more severe forms of the disease. In addition, spontaneous mutations may increase the risk of CMT occurring in future generations of a family.

The bottom line is that anybody can develop CMT, even if there isn't a family history of the condition.

What Are the Complications of CMT Disease?

Bone fractures

The most common complication of this disease is bone fractures. As the disease progresses, the bones in the feet and legs become weak and thin. This can lead to fractures, even with minimal trauma. In addition, the decreased sensation in the feet and legs can make it difficult to detect an injury, increasing the risk of fracture.

The Charcot-Marie-Tooth disease can also cause joint deformities, which can put additional stress on the bones and lead to fractures. Treatment for this complication typically includes immobilization, physical therapy, and surgery. However, in severe cases, amputation may be necessary.

Muscle cramps

One potential complication of Charcot-Marie-Tooth Disease is muscle cramps. Muscle cramps are involuntary, often painful contractions of the muscles. They can occur in any muscle but are most common in the legs.

The precise cause of muscle cramps is not known, but they may be associated with dehydration, electrolyte imbalances, or nerve damage. Treatment for muscle cramps typically involves stretches and massages. More severe cases may require medication or surgery. If you experience muscle cramps, it is important to see a doctor to rule out other potential causes.

Joint deformities

One of the most common complications associated with Charcot-Marie-Tooth disease is joint deformities. As the condition progresses, the muscles in the feet and legs gradually weaken. This can lead to changes in the way that the joints line up, resulting in deformities such as hammertoes, claw toes, and high arches. Joint deformities can cause pain and make it difficult to walk or stand for long periods. In severe cases, joint deformities may require surgery to correct.

Digestive problems

One of the complications of Charcot-Marie-Tooth disease is digestive problems. The most common symptom is constipation, which can be caused by damage to the nerves that control the muscles in the digestive system. This can lead to a build-up of waste in the intestines, which can be painful and uncomfortable. In severe cases, constipation can lead to bowel obstruction, which can be life-threatening.

Another potential complication is gastroesophageal reflux disease (GERD). This occurs when stomach acid leaks back up into the esophagus, causing pain and irritation. GERD can also lead to serious complications such as ulcers and Barrett's esophagus. Fortunately, there are treatments available for both constipation and GERD. However, it is important to see a doctor if you experience any symptoms of these complications.

Depression

People with CMT may feel isolated and anxious due to their chronic pain and disability. In addition, CMT can be difficult to diagnose, and many people with the disorder are not aware of the resources and support available to them. If you or someone you know has CMT, it is important to be aware of the potential for depression and seek help if necessary.

Foot ulcers

Foot ulcers are a common complication of Charcot-Marie-Tooth disease. The condition results in nerve damage and loss of sensation in the feet. This can lead to repeated trauma to the feet, which can eventually result in ulceration.

Treatment of foot ulcers typically involves offloading the pressure from the ulcerated area. This can be done with special shoes or braces that redistribute weight away from the ulcer. In some cases, surgery may also be necessary to remove dead tissue or to correct any underlying bone deformities. With proper treatment, most foot ulcers will eventually heal.

However, recurrent ulceration is a serious complication that can lead to amputation. Therefore, people with Charcot-Marie-Tooth disease need to be vigilant about monitoring their feet for early signs of ulceration.

How to Manage Charcot-Marie-Tooth Disease Through Diet and Nutrition?

One way to help manage the symptoms of CMT is through diet and nutrition. Certain foods can help improve muscle strength and function, and some foods can help improve nerve function. By including anti-inflammatory foods in your diet and the following nutrients in your diet, you can help manage the symptoms of CMT.

Foods to Eat

Anti-inflammatory foods

Inflammation can worsen CMT symptoms. Inflammatory cytokines are elevated in the blood of CMT patients. These cytokines can damage myelin, the protective sheath that surrounds nerve fibers. This damage can lead to loss of nerve function and muscle weakness. Including anti-inflammatory foods in your diet may help to reduce your risk of CMT or improve your symptoms if you already have the condition.

Anti-inflammatory foods are rich in antioxidants and omega-3 fatty acids. Some examples of anti-inflammatory foods include:

- blueberries
- brussels sprouts
- spinach

Omega-3 fatty acids

Omega-3 fatty acids are essential nutrients that are important for brain health and nervous system function. They are also anti-inflammatory, which can help to reduce inflammation throughout the body. In CMT, omega-3 fatty acids may help to reduce nerve damage. Therefore, including foods that are rich in omega-3 fatty acids in your diet may help to prevent or reduce nerve damage. Omega-3 fatty acid-rich foods include:

- oily fish, such as salmon and mackerel
- flaxseeds
- chia seeds

Antioxidant-rich foods

Antioxidants help to protect cells from damage. In CMT, antioxidants may help to protect nerve cells from damage. Including foods that are rich in antioxidants in your diet may help to prevent or reduce nerve damage. Antioxidant-rich foods include:

- fruits, such as berries and cherries

- vegetables, such as kale and broccoli
- tea

Nutrients that are important for nerve function

Nerve cells need certain nutrients to function properly. These nutrients include vitamins B12, vitamin D, Magnesium, Potassium, Calcium, Folate, and Zinc. Including foods that are rich in these nutrients in your diet may help to prevent or reduce nerve damage.

Vitamin B12

This vitamin is important for nerve health and can help to prevent nerve damage. Vitamin B12 helps the body to produce myelin, a substance that protects nerves from damage. Without enough vitamin B12, myelin production decreases, leading to nerve damage. Therefore, including foods that are rich in vitamin B12 in your diet may help to prevent or reduce nerve damage in CMT. Vitamin B12 is found in:

- meat
- poultry
- fish
- eggs
- dairy products

Vitamin D

Vitamin D is an essential nutrient that helps the body to absorb calcium. Calcium is important for bone health and muscle function. Vitamin D deficiency has been linked to muscle weakness, fatigue, and bone loss. In CMT, vitamin D deficiency may contribute to muscle weakness and problems with balance. Therefore, including foods that are rich in vitamin D in your diet may help to prevent or reduce these symptoms. Vitamin D is found in:

- oily fish, such as salmon and mackerel
- eggs
- mushrooms

You can also get vitamin D from sunlight. However, if you have CMT, you should avoid unprotected exposure to sunlight, as this can worsen your symptoms.

Magnesium

Magnesium is an essential mineral that is involved in over 300 biochemical reactions in the body. This mineral is important for muscle function, nerve function, and energy production. Magnesium deficiency has been linked to muscle weakness, fatigue, and problems with balance. In CMT, magnesium deficiency may contribute to muscle weakness and problems with coordination. Therefore, including foods that are rich in magnesium in your diet may help to prevent or reduce these symptoms. Magnesium-rich foods include:

- dark leafy greens
- nuts
- seeds
- whole grains

Potassium

Potassium is an essential mineral that helps to regulate blood pressure and heart function. It is also important for muscle function and nerve function. Potassium deficiency has been linked to muscle weakness, fatigue, and problems with balance. In CMT, potassium deficiency may contribute to muscle weakness and problems with coordination. Therefore, including foods that are rich in potassium in your diet may help to prevent or reduce these symptoms. Potassium-rich foods include:

- bananas
- sweet potatoes
- beans

Calcium

Calcium is an essential mineral that is important for bone health and muscle function. calcium helps the body to produce myelin, a substance that protects nerves from damage. In CMT, calcium deficiency may contribute to nerve damage. Therefore, including foods that are rich in calcium in your diet may help to prevent or reduce nerve damage. Calcium-rich foods include:

- dairy products
- leafy greens
- tofu

Folate

Folate is an essential nutrient that is important for cell growth and development. It is also important for the production of myelin, a substance that protects nerves from damage. In CMT, folate deficiency may contribute to nerve damage. Therefore, including foods that are rich in folate in your diet may help to prevent or reduce nerve damage. Folate-rich foods include:

- leafy greens
- beans
- nuts

Zinc

Zinc is an essential mineral that is important for cell growth and development, wound healing, and the immune system. In CMT, zinc deficiency may contribute to nerve damage. Therefore, including foods that are rich in zinc in your diet may help to prevent or reduce nerve damage. Zinc-rich foods include:

- beef
- chicken
- lobster

You can help avoid or lessen the symptoms of Charcot-Marie-Tooth disease (CMT) by maintaining a healthy diet and making nutritious food choices. However, to confirm that these adjustments are appropriate for your needs, you want to discuss them with either your primary care physician or a trained dietitian.

Foods to Avoid

Some foods may worsen the symptoms of CMT or interact with medications used to treat the condition. These include:

Processed foods

These foods are often high in sugar and unhealthy fats, which can contribute to obesity and insulin resistance. In addition, processed foods are often low in essential nutrients, including vitamin B12. This vitamin is important for nerve function, and a deficiency can lead to further nerve damage in people with CMT. As a result, avoiding processed foods is an important part of managing CMT.

Alcohol

Alcohol consumption can increase the risk of nerve damage. For people with Charcot-Marie-Tooth, this means that drinking alcohol may worsen their symptoms. If you have the disease, it is important to talk to your doctor about whether or not you should drink alcohol.

Caffeine

Caffeine can worsen the symptoms of CMT by causing the nerves to become more irritable and by increasing muscle twitching. In addition, caffeine can interfere with sleep, which is important for people with CMT as it helps to reduce fatigue and pain. As a result, people with CMT should avoid or limit their intake of caffeine-containing foods and beverages.

Sugar

Sugar has long been known to be detrimental to one's health. Consuming too much sugar can lead to several health problems, including obesity, heart disease, and diabetes. People with Charcot-Marie-Tooth disease are typically advised to avoid sugar as it can worsen their symptoms

If you have CMT, you should avoid or limit your intake of these substances. You should also avoid or limit your intake of processed foods, as they may contain ingredients that can worsen the symptoms of CMT.

Sample Recipes

Vegan Caribbean Bowl

Ingredients:

- 1 cup jasmine rice
- 1 cup coconut milk
- 1 cup broth
- 1 tsp. salt
- 1/4 cup unsweetened dried coconut flakes, shredded
- 4 leaves kale or collard greens, stems removed and sliced thinly
- 1/4 white cabbage, shredded
- 1/2 red bell pepper, julienned
- 1 lime, halved
- 1 tbsp. coconut oil
- 1/2 orange
- Optional: 1-2 tsp. sesame oil
- Optional, choices for garnish: avocado, carrot, cilantro lime, orange, pineapple, and/or scallion, may be combined or not

Marinade:

- 1/2 cup fresh squeezed orange juice
- 1/4 cup soy sauce
- 1 tbsp. jerk seasoning
- 1 tsp. toasted sesame oil (Asian variety)
- tempeh, cubed or sliced (may also use other protein sources if desired)

Instructions:

For the marinade:

1. Mix all the marinade ingredients.
2. Throw in the tempeh in the marinade. Let it soak for at least half an hour.
3. In a saucepan, pour in the rice, coconut milk, broth, coconut flakes, and salt.
4. Set to medium-high heat and leave to boil.
5. Lower heat and allow to simmer for about 20 minutes, covered.
6. Once done, turn off the heat and leave the rice for now.
7. In a bowl, put red pepper, kale, and cabbage. Squeeze half a lime over.
8. In a pan placed over medium-high heat, pour in coconut oil.
9. Add the marinated tempeh to the hot oil. Cook until all sides are cooked well.
10. Add a teaspoon or two of sesame oil if desired. Squeeze in half an orange.
11. Remove tempeh from the pan.
12. In a serving bowl, scoop in rice, tempeh, and vegetables.
13. Upon serving, garnish according to your preference.

Baked Flounder

Ingredients:

- 1 lb. flounder, filleted
- 1/4 tsp. salt
- 1 cup halved red grapes
- 1 tbsp. extra-virgin olive oil
- 2 tbsp. parsley, chopped finely
- 1 tbsp. lemon juice
- 1 cup almonds, chopped and toasted
- freshly ground black pepper, to taste

Instructions:

1. Preheat the oven to 375°F.
2. Place fish on a sheet tray. Season with olive oil, salt, and pepper.
3. Combine the almonds, grapes, lemon juice, parsley, 1-1/2 tsp. of olive oil, 1/8 tsp of salt, and black pepper in a bowl.
4. Bake the fish for about 3 minutes.
5. Flip the fish and return it to the oven.
6. Bake for another 3 minutes, or until the fish is starting to flake, while the center is still translucent. Don't overcook.
7. Serve immediately, topped with the grape mixture.

Salmon with Avocados and Brussels Sprouts

Ingredients:

- 2 lbs. of salmon filet, divided into 4 pieces
- 1 tsp. ground cumin
- 1 tsp. onion powder
- 1 tsp. paprika powder
- 1/2 tsp. garlic powder
- 1 tsp. chili powder
- Himalayan sea salt
- black pepper, freshly grounded

Avocado sauce:

- 2 chopped avocados
- 1 lime, squeezed for the juice
- 1 tbsp. extra-virgin olive oil
- 1 tbsp. fresh minced cilantro
- 1 diced small red onion
- 1 minced garlic clove
- Himalayan sea salt to taste
- black pepper, freshly ground

Brussels sprouts:

- 3 lbs. of Brussels Sprouts
- 1/2 cup raw honey
- 1/2 cup balsamic vinegar
- 1/2 cup melted coconut oil

- 1 cup dried cranberries
- Himalayan sea salt
- black pepper, freshly ground

Instructions:

To make the salmon and avocado sauce:

1. Combine cumin, onion, chili powder, garlic, and paprika seasoned with salt and pepper. Mix well before dry rubbing on the salmon.
2. Place the salmon in the fridge for 30 minutes.
3. Preheat the grill.
4. In a bowl, mash avocado until the texture becomes smooth. Pour in all the remaining ingredients and mix thoroughly.
5. Grill salmon for 5 minutes on each side or until cooked.
6. Drizzle avocado on cooked salmon.

To make the Brussel Sprout:

1. Preheat the oven to 375℉.
2. Mix Brussels sprouts with coconut oil. Season with salt and pepper.
3. Place vegetables on a baking sheet and roast for about 30 minutes.

4. In a separate pan, combine vinegar and honey.
5. Simmer in slow heat until it boils and thickens.
6. Drizzle them on top of the Brussels Sprouts.
7. Serve with the salmon.

Kale Fried Rice

Ingredients:

- 2 tbsp. coconut oil
- 2 whole eggs
- 2 large garlic cloves, minced
- 3 large green onions, thinly sliced
- 1 cup of carrots, cut into matchsticks
- 1 cup of Brussels sprouts, diced
- 1 medium bunch of kale, ribs removed and the leaves shredded
- 2 cups brown rice, cooked and cooled
- 1/4 tsp. Himalayan salt
- 1/4 cup of lemon balm leaves, diced
- 3/4 cups of shredded coconut, unsweetened variety
- fresh cilantro, for garnishing

Instructions:

1. Heat up a teaspoon of oil in a large skillet over medium-high heat.
2. Pour in the egg mixture.
3. Cook the eggs while occasionally stirring.
4. Remove from the pan and set aside.
5. Pour another teaspoon of coconut oil into the pan, along with Brussels sprouts, carrots, garlic, and green onions.

6. Stir every now and then until the vegetables look tender.
7. Add kale and salt.
8. Remove from the pan and put them into where the egg is.
9. Put the remaining coconut oil into the pan. Add in coconut flakes, stirring frequently
10. Add rice and stir it in.
11. Add the egg and vegetable mixture to the pan, as well as the lemon balm leaves.
12. Stir to combine and heat through.
13. Transfer to a serving bowl and garnish with fresh cilantro.
14. Serve and enjoy.

Asian-Themed Macrobiotic Bowl

Ingredients:

- 2 cups cooked quinoa
- 4 carrots
- 1 package of smoked tofu
- 1 tbsp. nutritional yeast
- 2 tbsp. coconut aminos
- 4 tbsp. sunflower sprouts
- 2 tbsp. fermented vegetables
- 1 cup of shiitake mushrooms
- 1 avocado
- 2 tbsp. hemp seeds
- 2-3 cooked beets
- coconut oil cooking spray

Dressing:

- 2 tbsp. miso paste
- 1 tbsp. tahini
- 1 clove garlic, crushed
- 1 tbsp. olive oil
- 1/2 lime, juiced
- 3 tbsp. water

Instructions:

1. Roast the carrots in the oven at 400°F for 30-40 minutes.

2. Wash the vegetables, trim, and spray them with coconut oil.
3. Add them to the oven. When they are cooked, set them aside till you are ready to assemble the Buddha bowl.
4. Make the dressing by combining all of the ingredients in a medium-sized bowl. If the dressing appears lumpy, add more water.
5. To build the bowl, put the quinoa on the bottom and then arrange the vegetables on top.
6. Sprinkle the bowls with hemp seeds and drizzle the dressing over top.
7. Now serve and enjoy!

Chicken Salad

Ingredients:

- 1 small can premium chunk chicken breast packed in water
- 1 stalk celery, large, finely chopped
- 1/4 cup reduced-fat mayonnaise
- 4 romaine leaves or red leaf lettuce, washed and trimmed
- 2 oz. blue cheese, crumbled
- 8 pcs. cherry tomatoes or 1 ripe tomato, quartered
- 1 cucumber, small and sliced thinly

Instructions:

1. Drain canned chicken and transfer to a bowl.
2. Put in celery and mayonnaise.
3. Mix lightly. Don't crush the chicken.
4. In a separate shallow bowl, place the lettuce neatly.
5. Add the chicken salad in the middle and sprinkle blue cheese over it.
6. Add tomatoes and cucumber slices to the plate.
7. Refrigerate before serving, cover with plastic wrap.

Baked Salmon

Ingredients:

- 2 salmon fillets
- 6 cups of fresh spinach
- 2 tsp. coconut oil
- 1/4 tsp. garlic powder
- 1/4 tsp. turmeric
- 3 large cloves of garlic
- lemon juice
- salt
- pepper

Instructions:

1. Preheat the oven to 400°F.
2. Line a baking dish with parchment paper.
3. Marinate salmon fillets in lemon juice, coconut oil, garlic powder, turmeric, salt, and pepper.
4. Let it sit for a few minutes. This may also be done the night before to help the juices and flavor get into the salmon.
5. Once the oven is ready, bake salmon for 15 minutes.
6. Cook some of the garlic in a pan with coconut oil.
7. Add spinach and cook until ready. Season with salt and pepper to taste.
8. Take salmon out of the oven and put spinach beside it.
9. Serve and enjoy.

Asian Zucchini Salad

Ingredients:

- 1 medium zucchini, sliced thinly into spirals
- 1/3 cup rice vinegar
- 3/4 cup avocado oil
- 1 cup sunflower seeds, shells removed
- 1 lb. cabbage, shredded
- 1 tsp. stevia drops
- 1 cup almonds, sliced

Instructions:

1. Cut the zucchini spirals into smaller parts. Set aside.
2. Put almonds, sunflower seeds, and cabbage in a large bowl. Combine the ingredients well.
3. Add zucchini to the mixture.
4. In a small bowl, mix vinegar, stevia, and oil using a whisk or fork.
5. Pour the vinegar mixture all over the zucchini mixture. Toss well. Make sure everything is covered with the dressing.
6. Refrigerate for 2 hours before serving.

Low FODMAP Burger

Ingredients:

- 1-1/4 lbs. ground pork
- 1/4 tsp. allspice
- 1/2 tsp. salt
- 1/2 tsp. white pepper
- 1/2 tsp. ground nutmeg
- 1/2 tsp. caraway seeds
- 1/2 tsp. ground ginger

Instructions:

1. Preheat the grill then prepare the patty.
2. Using a small mixing bowl, stir together the salt, pepper, allspice, nutmeg, and ginger until fully combined.
3. Place the ground in a large mixing bowl and add the spice mixture.
4. Mix thoroughly until spices are evenly distributed to the pork.
5. Make round, flat burger patties using the palm of your hands.
6. Grill the patties and serve with gluten-free buns and mustard sauce.

Stir-Fried Cabbage and Apples

Ingredients:

- 1 shallot, thinly sliced
- 1/2 apple, cut into cubes
- 1/4 savoy cabbage, sliced thinly into strips
- 3–4 radishes, sliced thinly
- 1/2–1 tsp. coconut oil
- salt, to taste

Instructions:

1. 1. Pour some coconut oil into a wok.
2. 2. Add shallot and cook until translucent.
3. 3. Add the cabbage, radish, and apples to the wok.
4. 4. Stir-fry for about 5 minutes. Don't overcook.
5. 5. Add salt to taste.
6. 6. Serve while warm.

Asparagus and Greens Salad with Tahini and Poppy Seed Dressing

Ingredients:

- 10 to 12 asparagus stalks, washed well and sliced into ribbons
- 5 radishes, washed well, and sliced thinly
- 2 to 3 rainbow carrots, peeled and sliced thinly
- 1 handful of wild spinach
- 1 small handful of microgreens, washed well
- 1 small handful of sunflower greens, washed well
- optional: a few pieces of chive blossoms

For the dressing:

- 2 tbsp. tahini
- 1 tbsp. poppy seeds
- 1 tbsp. extra-virgin olive oil
- salt
- pepper

Instructions:

1. For the dressing, whisk ingredients together in a small bowl.
2. In a separate bowl, toss salad ingredients into the mixture.
3. Drizzle dressing on salad upon serving.

Stir-Fried Cabbage and Apples

Ingredients:

- 1 shallot, thinly sliced
- 1/2 apple, cut into cubes
- 1/4 savoy cabbage, sliced thinly into strips
- 3–4 radishes, sliced thinly
- 1/2–1 tsp. coconut oil
- salt, to taste

Instructions:

1. Pour some coconut oil into a wok.
2. Add shallot and cook until translucent.
3. Add the cabbage, radish, and apples to the wok.
4. Stir-fry for about 5 minutes. Don't overcook.
5. Add salt to taste.
6. Serve while warm.

Managing CMT Through Lifestyle and Natural Methods

It is important to take an active role in managing CMT. Many different methods can be used including:

Exercise

Exercise is an important part of managing CMT. Exercise can help to preserve muscle mass, maintain joint function, and reduce pain. It is important to consult with a physical therapist or other healthcare professional before starting an exercise program.

Range of motion exercises

These exercises can help to maintain joint function and flexibility.

Strengthening exercises

These exercises can help to maintain muscle mass and prevent weakness.

Aerobic exercises

These exercises can help to improve endurance and reduce fatigue.

Physical therapy

Physical therapy can help to strengthen muscles and improve flexibility. It can also help to reduce pain and improve circulation. In addition, physical therapy can help to prevent further damage to the nerves. For these reasons, physical therapy is often recommended for people with CMT. However, it is important to talk to a doctor before starting any new treatment. With the right approach, physical therapy can be an effective way to manage CMT.

Occupational therapy

Occupational therapy can help people with CMT learn how to cope with the limitations of the condition. Occupational therapists use a variety of techniques to help patients manage their pain. For example, they may teach patients how to use proper body mechanics when performing tasks. They may also recommend specific exercises to help stretch and strengthen muscles.

In addition, occupational therapists can provide patients with tools and devices to help make daily tasks easier. By using a multifaceted approach, occupational therapists can help patients with CMT live fuller, more active lives.

Conclusion

CMT is a degenerative neurological condition that can cause muscle weakness and wasting, as well as numbness and tingling in the extremities. Although there is no cure for CMT, there are a variety of treatments that can help people manage the symptoms of the condition.

Exercise, physical therapy, and occupational therapy can all help to improve the function of muscles and reduce pain. In addition, people with CMT should eat a healthy diet and avoid cigarettes and excessive alcohol consumption. With proper management, people with CMT can live relatively normal lives.

If you or someone you know has been diagnosed with CMT, the Charcot-Marie-Tooth Association can provide you with information and resources to help you cope with the condition.

FAQ About Charcot-Marie-Tooth Disease

1. What is Charcot-Marie-Tooth disease?

Charcot-Marie-Tooth disease (CMT) is a progressive disorder that causes muscle weakness and atrophy in the hands and feet.

2. What are the symptoms of Charcot-Marie-Tooth disease?

The symptoms of CMT vary from person to person. Some people only experience mild symptoms, while others may have more severe symptoms. Symptoms of CMT can include:

- Muscle weakness
- Muscle atrophy
- Numbness and tingling in the hands and feet
- Pain in the hands and feet
- Loss of coordination
- Difficulty walking

3. What causes Charcot-Marie-Tooth disease?

CMT is caused by a mutation in one of several genes that are responsible for nerve function. These mutations can be inherited from a person's parents or they can occur spontaneously.

4. How is Charcot-Marie-Tooth disease diagnosed?

CMT is typically diagnosed by a neurologist. A diagnosis of CMT is usually made based on the symptoms a person is experiencing and their family medical history.

5. Can diet and nutrition help people with Charcot-Marie-Tooth disease?

Diet and nutrition play an important role in managing the symptoms of CMT. People with CMT should eat anti-inflammatory foods and foods with essential vitamins that help to ease nerve pain. It is also best to avoid pro-inflammatory foods that can make symptoms worse.

6. What are the complications of Charcot-Marie-Tooth disease?

Complications of CMT can include:

- Bone fractures
- Muscle cramps
- Joint deformities

- Digestive problems
- Depression
- Anxiety
- Foot ulcers

References and Helpful Links

Charcot-Marie-Tooth Disease (CMT)—Diseases. (2015, December 17). Muscular Dystrophy Association. https://www.mda.org/disease/charcot-marie-tooth.

Charcot-Marie-Tooth Disease Fact Sheet | National Institute of Neurological Disorders and Stroke. (n.d.). Retrieved September 28, 2022, from https://www.ninds.nih.gov/charcot-marie-tooth-disease-fact-sheet.

ePainAssist, T. (2019, August 16). What to Eat & Avoid When You Have Charcot Marie Tooth? ePainAssist. https://www.epainassist.com/diet-and-nutrition/what-to-eat-and-avoid-when-you-have-charcot-marie-tooth.

Lee, Y. (n.d.). Adjusting My Diet to Better Manage Cmt—Charcot-Marie-Tooth News. Retrieved September 28, 2022, from https://charcot-marie-toothnews.com/columns/diet-symptoms-ingredients/.

Mayo Foundation for Medical Education and Research. (2021, February 24). Charcot-Marie-Tooth disease. Mayo Clinic. Retrieved September 28, 2022, from https://www.mayoclinic.org/diseases-conditions/charcot-marie-tooth-disease/diagnosis-treatment/drc-20350522.

PhD, L. F. (n.d.). Charcot-Marie-Tooth and Diet—Charcot-Marie-Tooth News. Retrieved September 28, 2022, from https://charcot-marie-toothnews.com/charcot-marie-tooth-and-diet/.

www.ingramcontent.com/pod-product-compliance
Lightning Source LLC
LaVergne TN
LVHW051924060526
838201LV00062B/4671